MW01264910

Gastric Bypass Surgery

The Psychological Journey

by

Ranesa McNally. LCSW-C

authorHOUSE®

AuthorHouse™
1663 Liberty Drive, Suite 200
Bloomington, IN 47403
www.authorhouse.com
Phone: 1-800-839-8640

First published by AuthorHouse 8/14/2008

ISBN: 978-1-4343-7411-0 (sc)

Library of Congress Control Number: 2008907392

Printed in the United States of America
Bloomington, Indiana

This book is printed on acid-free paper.

This book is dedicated to:

My father, who always told me I could be anything I wanted to be, and actually meant it.

My family and friends, for without their love an support, I could never have come so far on my own journey.

And …

The Baltimore Bariatric Center, in particular Dr. William J. Roe, Jr. Dr. Roe continues to inspire me as well as countless hundreds of others as we find our way to a path of better health.

Preface

I began this book exactly two weeks after my father died of a sudden heart attack. After the shock passed, I realized there were many things I had been putting off. Events such as death often prompt us to start taking a look at our own mortality, doing things we thought could wait. Although I had been contemplating beginning this venture for quite some time, I became compelled by the "not putting off tomorrow what can be done today" mentality and recognized now is the time to put the thought into action. Much like the notion of undergoing gastric bypass surgery. You think about it, talk about it, and usually some small or large event makes you act on the thought. Your gut instinct tells you that now is the time to make some drastic changes in your lifestyle. My intent with this book is to give both those contemplating surgery and those who have previously undergone the procedure some concrete idea of some emotional changes that have become common before and after the surgery. I have performed hundreds of psychosocial assessments for those preparing for surgery, in addition to seeing patients for issues related to adjusting to life after the gastric bypass procedure.

As a post-bariatric patient of five years, and also as a therapist, it has become clear the medical procedure of gastric bypass surgery far surpasses simply being an instrument to help people lose weight and become healthy physically. It is also an instrument that fundamentally changes one's outlook mentally. There is a reason that psychological evaluation is necessary before undergoing this procedure. Initially, it is important to understand where people are mentally prior to surgery regarding feeling depressed or anxious, if they suffer from an addiction, their reasons for contemplating the procedure, their long-term expectations of surgery, and of utmost importance, their relationship with food.

Those who succeed long term tend to be those individuals who fully understand that an entire lifestyle change is necessary; this is not as simple as changing eating habits. This also means looking at how food has played a part in one's upbringing, when exactly one began struggling with the weight, the social and cultural implications related to obesity, as well as the role food plays in social settings. Also to be examined is one's outlook regarding exercise, the ability to follow directions, and issues of control. Emotional eating patterns are to be examined, as well as specific triggers to poor eating habits.

Who would think that one procedure could potentially affect every aspect of your life? I know you might be thinking, "I'm the same person I always was or will be." *Wrong!* Your core values remain the same, but as I have experienced and seen firsthand, your view of yourself, and at times others, does change. Obesity limits you in so many aspects; it's a fact in the overall quality of life. Even those who report overall self-love and high self-esteem recognize that there are times they are simply limited in their activities and abilities due to the excess weight. Those who choose to admit this recognize they are viewed differently as a person at a healthy weight as opposed to the "fat person" in public and private settings. Expectations change both internally and externally. Couple this with any kind of unresolved psychological trauma, and the changes are exacerbated. The bad news is, the psychological effects after gastric bypass have long been overlooked. The good news is, the medical community is finally recognizing these changes and does admit long-term success not only depends on changing the way you eat, but also changing the way you think.

And so journey begins …

In the Beginning ...

Let me start by saying, I don't have all the answers. I do, however, have a pretty good idea of what led you to resorting to surgical intervention to assist you in your weight loss. It is probable that you have various health problems related to the excess weight. You are probably tired much of the time. You probably have difficulty with everyday activities such as tying your shoes, walking up steps without being short of breath, sitting comfortably in a booth at a restaurant or at the movies, and the list goes on. You have probably been stared at by strangers and called derogatory names by children. You want a better quality of life. Good for you! However, keep in mind that to get the better quality of life, there are changes to be made to your lifestyle. There are certain foods you need to limit or refrain from and supplements you must take for the rest of your life. In this process, you cannot avoid exercise. The simple equation to losing and keeping off the weight has not changed. You do need to continue to limit what you eat, coupled with exercise. This is not a quick fix to losing weight and keeping it off. It is intended to give you a fighting chance to improve your health. You have done your research (I hope) and know the benefits and risks. Bottom line, the benefits are plentiful, and there are risks associated with undergoing any surgery. It is important to weigh each and understand the decision to undergo the bypass procedure is not to be taken lightly. It is important to be prepared for all aspects of changes that can occur in your life. You need to start with getting in touch with yourself and your expectations.

The question that I suggest you ask yourself is this. *Do I know myself?* Do I know if I eat out of emotion, not out of hunger? Is food my best friend or my worst enemy? Do I know those foods I can refrain from and can I do it long term? No sugar, no carbs, no or low fat? Am I aware that some foods I will not be able to eat again because I will be ill or won't be able to digest them? Do I know the consequences of "a bite too much"? Do I currently have a bad habit of just not thinking about what I put into my mouth and as a result have become a mindless eater? Do I take the time to enjoy my food? Do I have a food addiction? Do I eat in secret? Do I binge eat? Do I feel excessive guilt if I eat a "bad" food? Do I have an obsession with the scale? Do I know how to do this forever?

In answering these questions, don't panic. Just take a look at how much you know about what is expected post-surgery and the way you currently eat. If you had not given these factors any thought prior to contemplating surgery, now is the time to do so. Take the time to ask questions of your potential surgeon. Talk to folks who have previously undergone the procedure. Look for online forums where people openly discuss their successes and challenges. Start thinking about changes you will need to make regarding food choices and beverage intake prior to surgery.

These questions are just the beginning of the list you should answer honestly with yourself *before* the procedure. I say answer honestly, because I know how desperate you are to get to a healthy weight. I really understand the frustration. I know it would be so much easier to say, " I just have a slow metabolism; I can be okay giving up any food. I really don't have issues with giving up control. No problem." The thing is, this is the exact thinking that brings people into my office after surgery.

You need to be painfully honest with yourself regarding all your issues around food. I know a percentage of you really don't eat much, just not enough of the good stuff. I do recognize that medication and various medical issues contribute to difficulty in losing weight. There are real reasons besides our eating habits that we have not been able to lose and keep weight off in the past. In addition to these reasons, we have to take responsibility for our part. Maybe we eat well most of the time, but for whatever reason are not active enough to burn off those calories. Maybe we are so frustrated we just are fed up with thinking about food. Maybe late-night snacking is the issue. All that matters is that you can look at all the reasons you have become obese and vow to change those factors that are in your control.

Also to consider before surgery is your relationship with exercise. It could be an outlet that you welcome or a physically painful reminder of your extra weight each time you try to get active. Are you someone who starts out excited with a new piece of equipment, only to find it in the corner of the basement with clothes strewn on it a month or six months later? Are you someone who really (sort of) likes exercise, but has trouble finding time fitting it in your day? Is there always something better to do? Are you someone who honestly hates exercise because you find it difficult to walk from one room to another, let alone walk a quarter of a mile (forget a mile)? If you suffer from arthritis or severe joint pain, most exercise is too painful. And for most morbidly obese people (sorry, that's the medical term), the thought of going to the gym and feeling vulnerable and exposed is out the question. And what about those people who really do exercise by walking and using the proper equipment but continue to feel defeated after the attempts do not yield results? Or worse, the pounds come off, only to come back later, so they give up exercise completely. And it's true, it is hard to get back into exercise once you stop.

So looking ahead, you need a plan. You need to again honestly admit your love, hate, or indifference to food and exercise. Bottom line, you must moderately exercise to keep your weight under control long term—not just to keep from becoming obnoxiously jiggly and wiggly (more on this later), but because you need to move. Your heart needs to work out. Your joints need to move. If you suffer from depression, short or long term, or another mood disorder, you need to exercise regularly to increase the release of endorphins to your brain that release the positive energy to lift your spirits and give you emotional balance. Thankfully, there are workouts for the most physically challenged, such as water aerobics and specific physical therapy exercises based on your medical needs. There is a whole host of medical research to back up all the benefits of exercise. I also know you already know the importance of exercise but that getting started is difficult and when you're obese, it's twice as difficult. It seems to take so much energy just to walk a little, let alone work up a sweat. So you may need some help getting yourself started, but please move. As always, talk to you primary doctor before you start any exercise program. Depending on your medical issues, you certainly don't want to hurt yourself when you're trying so hard to get healthy.

Now that you have decided that yes, you want to feel better physically, and yes, you really do under-stand you need to eat healthy and exercise, why else are you having the surgery? Really, why? The answers will be different for everyone. After you have exam-ined your own reasons, hopefully you are doing this to get healthy and add some years to your life. You may want to be active with your kids or grandkids. You may want to experience activities that you cannot physically take part in currently. These are all valid reasons to pursue this form of weight loss. On the other hand, let me give you some examples of why I caution certain patients to resolve some issues psychologically before surgery. I may even suggest some people rethink the surgery completely if these reasons are top on your priority list. A big one I hear is, "I want to save my marriage or relationship." Let me explain. If you are unhappy in your relationship, losing the weight will not "fix" it. Your problems in your relationship go much deeper than what you weigh. In fact, it appears that if a relationship is not solid and the significant other is not in support of the decision to pursue bariatric surgery, the relationships may likely deteriorate post-surgery. *Please evaluate your relationship with your partner before surgery.* If there are issues to be examined, do it. If your other half is unwilling to work through the issues, figure out if you can commit to surgery and the lifestyle changes without his or her support. If you evaluate your other supports, you can be quite successful. But be realistic going in. You need to let go of the illusion that a thinner you will make any relational issues disappear. Once you are honest with yourself, you can be assured you are committed to making changes for yourself and no one else. If you get stuck on pleasing others in this process, you are more likely to self-sabotage later. If the people in your life cannot support you and may hinder you, release them to the extent you can or at least get some extra support, either through a support group or through counseling.

Another reason I ask patients to further examine their issues before considering this surgery is a recent presence of an eating disorder, such as bulimia or binge eating. If you have serious issues related to food that compel you to purge after eating or your eating is out of control (i.e., you eat enormous amounts of food to self soothe), please *do not* proceed with the surgery. *You will cause serious harm to your body and could very possibly die!* When asked this question by a health care professional, be honest. These issues are generally related to a psychological trauma and individual/group counseling is necessary. Similarly, any emotional eating needs to be examined before surgery, such as food being used to decrease emotions such as depression, anxiety, stress, or anger. You must plan other ways to deal with these emotions besides using food. For many of us, food was used as a coping mechanism, so a new coping skill can be developed. If you choose to ignore emotional eating patterns, you may harm your body and more likely than not, gain the weight back over time. That's right, this procedure is only a tool; often people gain some weight back as they ignore healthy patterns and return to detrimental, poor eating habits. This surgery will not cure a compulsive eating habit.

If you do have an eating disorder or need help establishing healthy coping skills, seek help from a local therapist specializing in these issues. Various support groups can also be very effective in helping you to deal with issues related to food. Also to consider is rectifying the reasons why these disorders have become present, as related issues or people related to these issues may still be present in your life. It will be important to recognize barriers that may still be a factor after surgery so that you can deal with them effectively.

Although various psychological disorders seem more likely to coexist with morbid obesity, such as depression or anxiety disorders, other disorders, such as the presence of a personality disorder or chronic disorder such as schizophrenia, is a red flag that this particular procedure may not be effective long term. The reasoning behind this statement lies in one's ability to follow through with positive decision-making consistently when certain disorders are present. It is important that food not be used as a tool to manipulate others or be refused as often happens when one's mental health decompensates. This is not to say someone with a personality disorder or chronic mental health disorder cannot be successful post-surgery, only that the disorder needs to be monitored closely after surgery and consistently managed. Unfortunately, even with careful management, it is more likely than not that these conditions will deteriorate throughout one's lifetime, therefore making it difficult to stick with a regime for any length of time consistently on a daily basis.

I always consider one's expectations following surgery. Most people want to decrease their physical ailments and increase their quality of life. However, if a person seems more concerned with the amount of weight he or she will lose in relation to how he or she will look and be perceived by others, I ask more questions. One young woman was completely convinced she would go from a size twenty-two to a size ten and look so fabulous she would finally become "the popular one" in her crowd. She believed this would help her find a boyfriend. It was very important that she meet others' expectations and believed if she were thin she would finally be accepted. After some discussion regarding some common misconceptions regarding her self-worth and the possibility of excess skin after losing a large amount of weight, she quickly reconsidered if she was ready for such a procedure. This was one case where the person was not grounded regarding realistic outcomes, and further education was needed. It is so very important for you to evaluate your expectations post-surgery and explore with professionals the possibility of those expectations being met.

The final (false) reason people may choose the surgery is to finally gain control. We all want to control something. For many people weight is the one area in their lives that they have not been successful in maintaining control over. They have successful careers and relationships, but controlling what they eat eludes them. Initially, most people feel really great about the level of control they have after surgery. Your smaller stomach pouch allows you to eat very little, so yes, you have control in the beginning. But over time, you need to decide if you can maintain this control. If you drink when eating, you can eat more, thus, no control. If you want to eat at a buffet event, with all sorts of poor food choices, can you maintain control? If your family eats solids and you are still eating liquids, you have no control. You will always struggle with making the right choices regarding food. You will always have to decide when and what are the correct foods to eat. The temptations will always be there. It's okay. What you can control is following instructions through the process. Once you establish good eating habits, you need to continue them. This is where your control is challenged. Your doctor will give you specific instructions, and this is no time to buck the system. Recognize your need to have control and any issues you may have with those you see as "authority" figures. Often we feel other people are taking away our ability to control a situation or that we don't have the good sense to make the right decisions for ourselves. Regardless of whether this rational or not, we can become very stubborn and make decisions based on anger and resentment, not based on what is the healthy choice. That childlike mentality of "you can't tell me what to do" pops up, and we react in a way that is not in our best interest, as if there is a point to prove. Subconsciously, you may not even realize you have issues with those in authority roles. Recognize your doctor has the authority regarding what you are expected to do pre- and post-surgery. It is imperative you give up what you perceive as control and realize that in following directions, you are actually taking control back. This is a hard concept for some folks. If you really can't let go of being told what to do in your best interest, then this procedure is not for you. If you can, keep reading.

What Can I Expect?

Keep in mind these are only a few reasons to search for other alternatives to weight loss, and that no method is absolute. This journey is completely individualized regarding reasons to pursue bariatric surgery and the success long term varies regarding outcomes. Your most guarded thoughts and feelings must be examined and a resolve to change whatever part of your life may hinder your success is the essential key to long-term success. However, as anyone who has undergone this procedure will tell you, you really don't know how complicated this can be emotionally until you have experienced it.

So after much research and contemplation, you and your doctor have decided this surgery is right for you. You have a plan of action and are feeling excited and ready for the process to begin. You are aware of adjustments to be made prior to surgery. You have cut your portions, are choosing healthier foods, and have increased your water intake. You are practicing chewing your food slowly, have eliminated carbonated beverages from your diet, and have quit smoking to prepare for optimal health. You have spoken to your support systems about your needs after surgery. You are avoiding negative comments and are focused on the positive. You have arranged to take the proper time off work to recover. You are ready to begin your new adventure. Then, you become anxious.

You begin to eat in response to the thoughts of giving up foods you previously enjoyed, maybe even loved. You begin to really understand your lifestyle is drastically going to change. It is normal for people to get in "last meal mode" before surgery. This refers to eating high-calorie foods at your favorite restaurants prior to surgery. While this is a natural response to impending deprivation, please proceed with moderation. Many people attend that last happy hour and celebrate the end of their old ways of behaving. It is fine to acknowledge the changes; just do not go in to the surgery with an "all or none mentality." If you believe that all your "favorites" are forever out of reach, you may experience some low level of depression. Also, giving up previous social outings around food may be necessary, and people often begin to feel they might be disconnected with others after surgery. In addition, fears associated with the actual procedure start to creep up. All of this is normal, but you need to prepare to deal with these emotions.

To combat the anxiety, particularly the night before surgery, try some simple relaxation techniques. Take some deep breaths. I know, everyone says this. That's because it works. As you breathe in, fill your abdomen with air. Do not pull your stomach in. Count to three and exhale slowly. Your stomach and upper body should relax. It may feel foreign at first, but practice is key. You can also clear your mind. Close your eyes and picture a bright white spot. Focus on that spot as you breathe. Oh, did I mention to do this in a quiet spot? No phone ringing, TV in the background, or people or animals craving your attention. If it's a nice evening, sit outside. If it's humid, let a fan blow on you face. The goal is to feel comfortable and in control to decrease the fear and anxiety.

Progressive relaxation is another technique to release any negative emotion. Close your eyes, start at your toes, and squeeze. Count to three and release.

Do this technique the entire length of your body. Breathe in as you squeeze and exhale slowly. Release negative emotions as you feel each part of your body relax. This technique can be used whenever you feel stressed or anxious.

This may be the time to review all the reasons why you have elected to have gastric bypass surgery. This is the time to think about all the things you will now be able to experience post-surgery, some things for the first time or since childhood. If you have not already written down your hopes for experiences after surgery, now is the time. All of these things will be invaluable later in your journey. I also encourage you to write a farewell letter to your current relationship with food. You may think this sounds corny, but try it. Write about how the relationship started and when, perhaps in childhood or after the birth of a child, and how food represented something to you during that time. Write about how food has come to affect you emotionally and physically, both in the beginning and now as you prepare to focus on the relationship with food in a healthy way. Write about why the relationship needs to change and release the old connection with food. Tuck this away. Again, rereading this later may serve as a source of strength.

Finally, make sure you take a full-length picture of yourself. I know you hate pictures when you're heavy, but this will be the last "fat picture." Certainly pictures are not typically our friends, but this one will be one to look back on. Many doctors do this for patients prior to surgery at the last pre-operative visit. If not, take one at home.

You may choose to take a picture monthly after surgery for the first year, but this first one brings you back to why you are working so hard and keeping positive habits. This is the picture no one will believe is you. This is the picture about which you say, "That won't be me again." Years from now, you may not remember this person on the outside. Put this picture away and release this image for now. It is time to focus on a healthier you from this day forward.

You can expect all kinds of emotions before surgery, and definitely a whole new host of emotions after surgery. Most people describe their journey as a "roller coaster" of emotions, mostly positive, but oftentimes confusing in relation to adjusting to their new bodies. You would expect to feel elated all the time, but for most people, to lose some weight is not enough. It's the search for more: more weight loss, more acceptance, more activities, a better body image, off the charts self-esteem, etc. However, sometimes it is not that simple. It takes internal work to feel self-worth; it's more than what you look like on the outside. Although we have worked hard to lose the weight, it may never be enough for acceptance by some people. It's important that we learn to accept ourselves, not basing how we see ourselves on others' perceptions. Sometimes it takes losing the weight to begin to look at other areas we need to improve. This is perfectly normal, as long as you are aware of the work that lies ahead.

You may be thinking, "I know all this; this is not me." I need to tell you some of the most grounded individuals feel somewhat overwhelmed that they in fact are looking for more after losing the weight, and do feel some confused emotions regarding outcomes. We all like to think we have it all worked out, but recognize that if some of these thoughts and feelings do become present, it really is normal. Any large changes in your life are bound to throw you off center initially. Even though you may have not been happy with being overweight, it probably has been what you have known for many years, maybe most of your life. It will take some time to become accustomed to a thinner you and a different lifestyle, even when all the changes are good. Even those people who experience nothing but positive outcomes post-surgery in every aspect still need some time to let it all sink in. Just be aware that if all these changes feel foreign or a bit uncomfortable, it is to be expected.

Moving Right Along

The surgery is over and you are home. You are uncomfortable and tired. You are beginning your liquid diet. A few days into this and you have a routine. Suddenly, you smell food! Someone is cooking and it smells wonderful! Like nothing you have ever smelled before. Now, keep in mind, you have no appetite and prior to this smell or sight of real food, you had no desire to eat. But suddenly, *you are ravenous.* I assure you, it's all in your mind. Now you're angry. You are overcome with a desire to strangle whoever decided to cook. How dare they eat when you and your poor body are withering away on liquids! The nerve!

Hold it! Get a grip! This was your decision, and your rational mind realizes you cannot eat yet. You will be back in the hospital. You did not go through major surgery to freak out now. Take a breath. You really don't want to hurt the person who cooked. Hey, the rest of the family has to eat. You will eat too, all in good time. This is simply the first of many times you will be faced with not being able to eat what others eat. What you are experiencing is grief and loss related to food. Who knew? Now you understand what those people post-op were talking about. It is not uncommon to feel sad about not being able to enjoy food as you once did. This is simply a reaction to doing something different. In making changes, you are letting go of habits you have had for years. Good or bad, this was your way of doing things. At times, you may feel like it's unfair and wonder why you chose this route. So back to the list of why you had the surgery to begin with. This is normal, and you need to get grounded. You are simply in the first stage of retraining yourself to eat and think healthy. This is the time to get with some supports, in person or online. This is the time to realize you are not alone in this process and need to take advantage of others' encouragement. Most people say the first month post-op is the most difficult in terms of transition regarding food.

Now you refocus and get through the liquid, the purées, and the mushy foods. Finally, it's time to try some solid food. Some of you may be a little nervous about this. I know this sounds strange, but more than a few people worry (irrationally) that they may start to gain some weight back once they begin to eat solid foods again. This stems from years of yo-yo dieting. You spend so much time cutting back on whatever the "diet" says to cut, that as soon as you start to eat that item again, you gain the weight back. For many people, this is what leads to surgical intervention, as we have lost the ability to eat all things in moderation. So it makes sense people fear gaining the weight from eating. It also can be difficult after you see that large weight loss common after those first few weeks. It is not uncommon to drop twenty to thirty pounds the first month, as you have to have solid foods in this time. This fear can be harmful if it keeps you from following the proper protocol. You need to learn to eat again the proper way. This is the way to shed pounds and keep it off. I was able to lose 175 pounds and have fluctuated up or down ten pounds since losing the weight. This is a result of following directions and keeping positive habits. Not to say I haven't strayed from time to time, but I have learned that returning to eating healthy in controlled portions is the key to keeping it off. The whole point is to make lifestyle changes and eat healthy, not to drink your food for the rest of your life. I say this because many people get comfortable with the liquid protein. While this is essential in the beginning, it needs to be replaced with actual food when your doctor says you're ready. The goal is to eat small portions of healthy food. The goal is not to return to the hospital due to an irrational fear of gaining weight.

Another fear is getting sick or vomiting when eating. You body is learning to accept food again too. You may vomit initially, but don't get stuck. I know this sounds bad, because who likes this feeling, but it is likely to happen a few times. This is less likely if you take very small bites and chew, chew, chew. You will learn to tolerate most foods over time. Everyone is different in this stage, so experiment within reason as your doctor advises. Yes, fear the dumping syndrome. This occurs when you eat too much of foods high in sugar or fat. Some people dump on anything in excess. Really watch your intake of what we all call "bad" foods. If you know you need to stay away from sugar, do so. Find healthy substitutes. Same with those foods that contain fat. In this day and age, there are pretty good-tasting alternatives for most foods. Experiment until you find what works for you. Many people get comfortable with certain foods and try to stick with a routine once they learn what works. Having a set routine regarding when and what you are eating most days can also help with letting go of thinking about food all the time. This is a common complaint after surgery. People are so focused on what to eat or not eat, it can become obsessive. To some degree this is necessary, as you will always need to be aware of what you are eating. But, when it becomes all you think about, you need to relax a bit. If you have formed new habits, these habits will become less exhausting to follow through with each day. On the opposite side of this, some people need variety to feel satisfied. Whatever you need individually is fine, as long as food does not become all that you focus on. Use positive self talk, use your supports, but above all, you must eat!

Another factor that can be difficult for some people to let go of is the obsession with the scale. Although others may disagree, I have found overall that overuse of the scale can be a barrier as opposed to a motivator for weight loss. If you are eating properly, you will lose weight, so why weigh yourself every day? If you are seeing your doctor for monthly follow ups once a month, as most bariatric programs set up for the first year post-surgery, this will be sufficient for monitoring your progress. Your scale may differ from your doctor's scale, and many bariatric scales also measure body mass index as well. This is key, as it not only shows weight loss, but also fat loss. The numbers for fat loss are as important, if not more important, than actual pounds shed. BMI really shows how healthy you are. And let's face it, on any given day, your weight can slightly fluctuate due to water weight. This is not an old wives' tale. So if you constantly look at the numbers and they don't move or go up slightly, it can really deflate your motivation. Thus fear of failing (again) and anxiety can become present. Then old habits start to arise and *bam!* You gain some weight for real. If you are on the scale daily or several times per week, remove the scale immediately! The scale can become a trigger or excuse to eat (or not eat) as instructed and therefore is no good for you. For those of you craving control, this is a step in the right direction. You need to gain control by focusing on better habits and not allowing those numbers to control you. Every choice you make to get healthy is taking control. Let these choices be a driving force.

Let's talk about some other triggers that can hinder you progress, not necessarily right away but throughout the process. Our society generally uses food for celebrations, get-togethers, grieving, and for "just because" opportunities. As children, we learned to associate food with all the emotions related to all these occasions—happy, sad, and content. Also, many of us generally use food to bring people together. We meet friends for dinner, go to someone's home, or invite people to our home. Hey, and what about sports get-togethers? Superbowl parties and March madness are great excuses to overindulge. Don't forget the wedding showers, baby showers, birthday parities—the list is endless. All of these are triggers. Unless you are throwing the party, you don't have much say in what is being served. So you need to plan. You don't necessarily need to decline invitations; just be aware of foods that may be tempting. These events provide a way to rethink why we get together, and you can begin to focus on the people and friends involved instead of the food. You will learn to enjoy yourself in spite of the food, not because of the food. If you feel you cannot truly resist the temptations, make an appearance and keep the visit short, or bring a support along to help. Sit away from the food and ask a friend or spouse to fix your plate. Focus on the reason you are at the occasion and the people hosting the event. This may feel awkward at first, but the more you attend these events and go out with friends and family, the more comfortable you will become in adapting to various surroundings. In the beginning, be ready for people to ask questions about how little food you are eating. You really don't have to tell anyone anything if you choose not to at a social event. Tell them you're not really hungry and leave it at that. If they pressure you further, tell them you're watching your weight. This is perhaps the most uncomfortable time for very private people. You may not be able to avoid questions, but be prepared for a response.

The most stressful time for someone watching what he or she is eating happens around the holidays. Trying to keep balanced during these times can be quite a challenge. Holidays are always full of too much of everything, including food and family expectations. Also, let's not forget that many religions include access to foods specifically reserved for certain holidays. This is tough to ignore and twice as difficult if you have a "just take a bite" relative present at a function. Back to planning. You must have a conversation with those well-meaning relatives *before* the occasion. There is quite enough to deal with in family gatherings without feeling pressure to eat what you cannot or more than what you need to at someone else's prompting. If you don't have the opportunity to speak with a well-meaning relative, practice what you will say at his or her prompting for you to eat or comments about your weight loss. You may feel guilty or tempted, but planning ahead and knowing your limits will help. Practice saying, "It all looks delicious, but I really can't eat another bite." Say it with a smile. Remember, this is about taking care of you and no one else. Keep in mind, the first round of holidays may not be the most difficult, depending on when you had your surgery. It may not be until the following year that the food appears more tempting because you are able to eat a bit more. We all know everything there is to know about dieting, so back to basics. Eat some fruit or vegetables before attending an occasion, and drink plenty of water to assist with avoiding temptation. Also, practicing the two-minute rule may be helpful. When those thoughts creep up (and they will) to "just have one more bite" or "I'll just run through the fast-food joint for a quick burger, a few fries ..." whatever the temptation may be, you must remember you have a choice. Start the tape running in your head. If you can talk to yourself about all the reasons you don't need that extra bite of empty-calorie food for just two minutes, you can avoid a bad choice. The impulse will pass, and you can pass on that bite or drive right by that fast food joint. If you can keep up the talk about all the positive reasons to keep up your hard work for that two minutes, you can keep on track. The trick is to run this tape each time, and it can be a challenge. The more you practice, like anything else, the better you get at it. Instead of "I deserve this cookie," you need to say, "I deserve to feel well." You do deserve to treat yourself well, but not with a cookie. You deserve to feel great and be healthy. Know these thoughts will become more automatic and the old way of thinking will pass. Practice positive talk for two minutes every day, regardless of the presence of a trigger. Even if it feels silly at first, it does become more natural. If you give in and take a bite, don't let this be an excuse to take another bite. We are great at making small hurdles become huge obstacles. The months fly by, and suddenly external factors begin to take you off your stringent, well planned path. A family member becomes ill and demands your time. You decide to move, change jobs, the kids start acting out, you take on extra hours at work, and the list goes on. Suddenly, you don't quite make it to the gym; you forget that B-12 shot or supplement. The minute you recognize it, regardless of why, take a deep breath. Rearrange your plan. For example, if you need to be at home more often and really cannot make it to the gym as often as you would like, work out at home. If you can't bend as life changes, you may find that compulsion to self sabotage your efforts coming back. We can really get stuck on the, "Why do I keep self-sabotaging?" There could be a different reason for everyone. I know this sounds wishy-washy, but again, there are a million reasons why we make excuses. The trick is to change the pattern, regardless of the reason. I believe no one *wants* to stop doing positive things to become healthy, but it is hard work every day. This is not a "sometimes when I feel like it" deal, but you do need to let go of the perfectionism that you will make all the right choices and follow through each and every day. The perfectionism mentality will destroy your motivation and hard work. I don't know of one person, be it a fitness expert, a doctor, or a successful bariatric patient, who does not follow through at some time. Be gentle to yourself. This is a constant learning process. I have learned through trial and error, and sometimes situations beyond my control, that you just can't get it right all the time. If I get the flu, I really can't exercise and eat right. I remember the first time this happened. I panicked. All I could think was, what about the protein? I'm going to get fat because I can't work out. I really became obsessed. That's right, the therapist obsessed. Then, after I began to feel better, I had no desire to exercise. I craved comfort food. I literally forced myself to get on the treadmill. I gagged when I ate scrambled eggs. But I did it anyway. I thought, "You just spent three days worrying about what you could not do. What a waste of energy if you don't get back on track." I called a friend who was sympathetic but also gave me the kick in the pants I needed. It's easy to get others motivated, but difficult to do it for yourself. My friend held me accountable, and I persevered. And yes, these difficult times happen from time to time even now. However difficult, use your supports to overcome the negative thoughts.

It's all in the way you perceive the challenge. If you convince yourself this is too hard, it will be. If you allow one day of bad choices to dictate your progress, I guarantee the next day will be just as difficult. How much do you need to beat yourself up? If you learn from any experience, you are progressing. When you accept yourself and all your imperfections, you accept that you create success or failure. You wanted control; now it is yours.

All of this has been said simply to make you aware of the challenges, not to discourage your progress. I am a believer in "knowledge is power." If you are aware of what lies ahead, it is easier to plan a way to overcome the barriers. Most of the people who see me post surgery had little idea initially that all or some of these barriers mentioned could hinder their progress. Or the mentality was, "It won't be me." At the very least, people are surprised when barriers crop up. Most people are surprised at how vulnerable they feel after losing weight. They are not prepared for all the attention, at how people look at what you eat all the time, they way people appear to constantly be sizing you up. It can add up to a lot of pressure. You are doing so well and the pressure sets in. Just when you're on a roll, there it is; you are tempted. You just want to eat so people will leave you alone. Don't give in. For many just one bite of chocolate or sip of soda starts a downward spiral. Ask anyone who has had this surgery. Most people say if they had the opportunity, they would not have given in to temptation. However, we are human. The key is to set limits. A bite will not put on the weight, but several bites daily will. In all reality, for most of us, we did not become obese by avoiding the junk food and high-calorie drinks. Keep in mind sugar and bad carbohydrates *will* leave you chasing that higher sugar level all day. So often those carbohydrates and sugar lead to a negative pattern. If you get caught in the cycle, go back to basics. You will have a need to monitor you eating habits for the rest of your life. Remember the measures you took to get healthy, and dig out the pictures post-surgery. This can be very effective in jolting you to get back on track.

Then and Now

You need to get familiar with the genetic history and lifestyle patterns that have led you to where you are now. Let's look at your upbringing. I hear the same story over and over again, including my own. Family time revolved around food. "Clean your plate, people in other countries are starving" was heard at every meal. You could not throw away or leave food on your plate because you would be punished. This was a reality of childhood for many people. Maybe the entire family was overweight. Or more frustrating, you were the only overweight person in the family. Everyone else could eat whatever he or she wanted and stay thin. There are dozens of variations. Bottom line is, a combination of genetics and learned bad habits contributes to weight gain. Just don't let this make you get stuck. Many people have a hard time leaving food on their plates as adults or feel guilty for throwing away food. The way to handle this issue is to eat from a smaller plate and give leftover food to someone else (or even the dog) when you can. Whatever you do, do not overeat because there's food left on your plate. Initially, putting too much on your plate will happen all the time. Measure the portions. Listen to your body. Take your time eating. And by all means, get your mother's voice out of your head. No one will suffer if you leave food on your plate. However, you will suffer if you overeat.

Many people say they feel their parents used food to express love or to make sure they were healthy. Depending on the era your parents were brought up, they may not have had access to plentiful food and therefore showered you with food because they could. Maybe they did not limit what you ate. Maybe you grew up in the era of fast food. Maybe you did not gain weight until adulthood, making poor choices on the run and no longer being able to keep up with that younger metabolism. Whatever the case may be, it's important to look at patterns related to food and where they came from in order to break the cycle.

Speaking of mothers or other well-intentioned family and friends, recognize everyone around you is adjusting to the new you. At times those people who initially encouraged you may seem to be sending mixed messages. Mom may say you're getting too thin. She encourages you one day and brings you a piece of cake the next. Your sister suddenly develops an attitude that is not favorable toward you. Your close friend seems distant. The more you lose, the more different you look. So how come you look better and feel great and those people closest to you suddenly seem to make you feel emotionally worse than you did at your highest weight?

These folks worry that you are changing. In many ways you are. You have better self-esteem. You have more energy. You're not as available to some as you once were because you're busy *doing*, not being sedentary. Maybe prior to weight loss, you were the "smart one" and your sister or friend was the "pretty one." Now the roles have switched. Suddenly everyone you meet is noticing you. Of course, some of these changes may make you a little unnerved or anxious, but to those around you, you are now the competition (or so they think). Your weight loss may be bringing up all sorts of insecurities for other people. We like to think we don't have that much of an effect on others, but believe me, their reactions speak clearly. It will be important not to internalize negative reactions, which could lead you to feeling guilty and ultimately lead to self-sabotage. When you see others acting differently, do not ignore it. Have a conversation about what you see. Sometimes others don't even notice that they are treating you differently. Bring it to their attention and let them know you realize this is a difficult adjustment for them. Also, let them know how you are feeling during this time. They may be relieved to hear you're as uncomfortable as they are at times. Above all, let them know you need their support now more than ever.

This also goes for significant others. Chances are, they are really proud of you and are also really freaked out. We all hear the stories—you know, people get thin and their relationships fizzle. Please be assured, there was much more than weight that was going on in this relationship that caused it to end. It's normal that a significant other may feel insecure concerning your weight loss, but if he or she leaves you or you choose to leave after the weight comes off, something in this relationship is off! Love does not end because you look different; love ends because true emotions become evident. Maybe it's getting more self-confidence to face what is wrong, or maybe you won't be a doormat for someone else anymore. The reality is that if the relationship is a good one, the surgery and weight loss will make it better. You have more energy to do things together, sex is definitely different, but definitely better, and you give more emotionally and physically. Your job at this stage is to reassure those close to you that despite the changes you are going through, you will continue to be there for them, just as they have been there for you. The more time passes, the more comfortable your significant other becomes when he or she realizes you are still the same person who loves him or her as you always have been. Leave the lines of communication open and talk about whatever issues come up around these changes. This is the best defense to combat any feelings of vulnerability in your relationship.

Some very important people that are often overlooked in the process are the children in your life. Hopefully you explained, on an age-appropriate level, why you need this procedure. Be prepared for questions as you eat very little and begin to drop the weight. I have often heard children express their concern that their mom, dad, aunt, uncle, etc., is sick. They may not understand that a smaller you is a healthier you. I have also heard (quite alarmingly) among pre-adolescent and other adolescents struggling with their weight that they don't worry as much because they will "just have surgery when I'm older." Please address this issue if there are overweight children in your life. Even if they don't bring it up, be very specific as to all the health issues related to morbid obesity. Encourage them to eat healthier and exercise with you. They need to see firsthand the work needed to attain a healthy weight and maintain it, regardless of surgery. Usually once they see firsthand the procedure is not a magic bullet, they tend to put it in perspective. Kids are also a great motivator. You want to be a good role model, and they can be your biggest cheerleader. Also, when you want to eat something that is not great for you, just picture them, and the guilt will help you to stay on track.

Another area that is affected by your weight loss may be your work environment. If you work with people in any capacity, be assured people will wonder why you're out for recovery and why you are losing weight so quickly. It's up to you to decide when to inform your boss and/or co-workers about your decision to pursue gastric bypass surgery. The workplace is often full of gossip, true or not. You may have told some select coworkers about your decision to pursue surgery and requested their silence if asked by others you have not told. It is generally a good idea before surgery to keep those with negative opinions and naysayers in the dark. This is all well and good until you start dropping drastic amounts of weight quickly. Be prepared for questions, both out of concern and curiosity. If you've established supports on the job, that's wonderful. If not and most people don't know, you may want to share, if only to put a stop to rumors such as you're sick, you're having trouble a home, etc. People will create reasons why you're losing weight if you are not upfront. Another common occurrence is the boss's perception of work performance once you have lost some weight. If you have a physically demanding job, of course your performance will be better and much easier for you to perform. But ... how about those people who have always done a good job, but suddenly you're getting noticed for it, just because you're thinner? Ouch.

You really do notice in situations like this the *huge* bias (*Ha!*) society has concerning obesity. This can be touchy because it is extremely irritating to think you look more "socially acceptable" and therefore are afforded more opportunities in the work-place. So your dilemma here is whether to take the opportunities because you deserve them or allow your anger at how unfair (and it is) the situation is when your performance was never recognized when you were significantly overweight prevail. It depends on the whole picture. Do you like your job, co-workers, hours, etc.? Then, hey, it's just another perk. But … if you are already in a dissatisfying job or there is discord and unnecessary stress, then use this recognition to build your self-esteem and get the job of your dreams, somewhere else. Now that you have the stamina to give more to the job, don't give that energy to a job that does not deserve you. Many people choose this time to change careers or go back to school. Don't change what is not broken, but if you're unhappy or desire more from your work life, go for it!

Now you have all this energy and no idea what to do with it. Think back to that list of things you wanted to do after surgery but physically could not or would have been too embarrassed to try. Now is the time to start on this list. It could be something smaller like walking into a gym or something bigger, like scuba diving. You may be faced with not knowing what you want to do in place of watching TV or surfing the Internet. You may need to look at those things you enjoy and start getting some new hobbies. This process is about having a more fulfilling life. So check out all your options. This is also imperative as you learn to replace old coping skills with new ones.

If you used to snack while watching TV, what could be a better option to keep your hands busy? If your favorite activity was meeting friends for dinner, what else could you do when you get together? This takes some thought, and you may find you're not the one to go crazy with new activities, but need some low-key options to keep you busy and not so focused on eating. Regardless of your unique needs, as you find yourself able to do more, take advantage of it as you create new healthy outlets.

I would like to spend a little time discussing the inevitable issue of excess skin post-surgery. This can affect even those of us with overall positive self-esteem. Most people say that although they fell pretty good when they are dressed, they feel really bad after seeing the jiggly, loose skin when they are undressed. At times this can affect people feeling comfortable being intimate with their partner. What you need to remember is that you have lost a large amount of weight in a small amount if time. This is normal. The amount of excess skin varies individually depending on where you carry the majority of your weight and also your age post-surgery. Another factor is the resolve to exercise regularly post-surgery. Initially, I don't think most of us spend much time thinking about this because the weight loss is and should be most prominent. As the weight falls off that first year, most people complain of feeling uncomfortable about the amount of skin they see. Feeling self-conscious at this time is normal. The good news is, if you exercise regularly and give you body some time to tone up, much of the skin does bounce back in some cases. In other cases, regardless of the exercise, the skin is there. I was fairly young when I had surgery and unfortunately, despite my best efforts, I still had some skin. Certainly nowhere near what it was when I initially lost the weight, but it was there. You need to give exercise a chance before you consider removing the skin. I say this to prepare you for a decision to remove it if you can afford it, as often insurance does not cover these procedures, or learn to accept it. Keep in mind the procedures require a good deal of recovery time and are not easy processes. This is a very personal decision. At times it is necessary to have the skin removed due to developing rashes from the excess skin Oftentimes it's the desire to look better, generally not out of vanity, but out of feeling self conscious. Please don't misinterpret this or think that you will care about the skin at all. Just be aware it may be a factor in the process, and you need to be aware of your options. Before making any decisions about plastic surgery, research you surgeon thoroughly and make sure he or she has experience with bariatric patients. Examine all your options and make the best decision for you.

Body image will be a factor in this society, regardless of your weight. Instead of focusing on those areas you don't like, focus on those that you do. Take a look at the neck bone you now have. See the difference in your facial structure. Notice how you can see muscle where there was fat previously. Appreciate your total body for what it can now do for you. Your legs are stronger and help you walk or run without so much effort. Your heart is healthier and stronger. You have the ability to ride a bike, skate, and so much more. It takes far more work to begin to appreciate all those positive things about your body, and it takes away your focus on all the weight you have lost when you start to pick yourself apart. You will have to constantly challenge your thoughts when your negative self talk pops up. Refocusing your thoughts on those positive areas of your body and all that it is now capable of will help you to improve the way you view your body, wherever you're at in the process.

More on socializing. We touched on going out to dinner with friends, interactions with co-workers, and challenging others' perceptions. We have not really focused on how other people start to really notice you. Perhaps as a large person, you tried not to be noticed or to blend in. Nobody likes to be pointed out as the fattest person in the room. No one likes those pitiful stares or looks of disgust. But how do you deal with looks of interest? What do you do when people look at you in a great outfit or the opposite sex strikes up a conversation? Definitely great for your ego, but it may also bring some anxiety. Many people, single or married, have a difficult time accepting positive interest and a more challenging time knowing how to react. What do you say when a person who would never look at you twice before you lost the weight suddenly buys you a drink or asks if you're single? Do you get mad, embarrassed, or question that motive? Maybe all three. Admit it. As a large person, people love you for who you are, not your looks. I'm not saying obese people can't be attractive. Hey, I was one of them. I loved and still love myself regardless. But I am also not blind to how society as a whole views large people. It really is quite an interesting phenomenon. It is important to recognize where you stand on this issue and get comfortable with being uncomfortable for a while. It's important because some people allow these encounters to make them hide. Some people even start developing bad habits again in the hopes of avoiding being approached. Fear is the biggest motivator and the biggest threat for self-sabotage. If you begin to avoid social situations, you deprive yourself of some opportunities to meet some great people. Don't automatically throw daggers or assume they would not speak to you if you were heavy. Maybe you're more approachable now because you are more outgoing. Even if this is the case, so what? The point is you feel and look better and people do notice. Work on your self-esteem and take the interest as a compliment. This could be an opportunity to meet an interesting person. If the person turns out to be someone you are not interested in, how different is it that you can be the one, maybe for the first time, to say you're not interested? Maybe for the first time you will have the self-confidence to make this type of decision and not settle for someone less than you deserve. It could just be a game to see if you can get "the look." Whatever the situation, this is the time to deal with all of these emotions. No more hiding. It is time to say, "Hey, world, here I am."

A dilemma that appears to be common among men going through this process is not being identified as "the big guy," "Mr. Big," or whatever name they have been affectionately called previously. Some men I have worked with state that they identified with being "the big guy" and to some degree felt powerful being obese. After losing the weight, some men have difficulty redefining their role and say they actually miss being singled out, as they find at their normal weight they no longer stand out. This requires looking more at how they perceive themselves and redefining how others see them. Men have just as fragile self-esteem as females, so this is important to examine in order to not allow self-sabotage to creep up because you are suddenly feeling uncomfortable with your new body. This is the time to remember you are now at a healthy weight and need to maintain your weight loss in order to avoid medical issues in the future, which is the number one reason you chose to undergo surgical weight loss in the beginning of your journey. Never be deterred by external forces when it comes to making the right decisions regarding staying healthy.

Improving Your Quality of Life One Less Pound at a Time

There are so many benefits to this surgery to improve your health. There are also many, many ways this surgery improves your quality of life. These improvements drastically contribute to alleviating depressive symptoms related to obesity, decreasing anxiety, and phobias related to being overweight, and improves overall self-esteem and feelings of self-worth. It can be such an empowering and exciting time. Those who really can grasp the enormity of these changes are generally those morbidly obese people who have never had the everyday ease and experiences that those of average weight at some point in their lives have had. Those little everyday experiences are the best motivators to keep the weight off. For instance, being able to see your feet to tie your shoes with the bow in the middle! Taking a bath comfortably in the bathtub. Fitting in the booth in a restaurant. Going to the movies and sitting comfortably in the seats! Riding amusement park rides! Running around with kids and grandkids. Woo-hoo! The list goes on and on as you lose weight. Each experience is to be remembered and never taken for granted. Remember, those who have never been obese may not appreciate your newfound freedoms. I remember the first time I ran up the steps without being short of breath. I was so excited I called my husband. He seemed a bit confused. It was then I realized he really did not know how it felt to enjoy everyday activities after being deprived for so long. I spent some time explaining just walking around was easier, let alone actually participating in activities. Those closest to us may support us, but may truly not understand the excitement we now experience from everyday activities most people take for granted. This is the reason support groups or contact with other bariatric patients is so important to your mental health. You need other people to know what you are feeling and those who can relate to those feelings. Celebrating the small hurdles as you progress in the process is just as important as initially losing the weight. You don't want to just lose it; you want to keep it off. All of these experiences are the things you build on as you live a more productive quality of life.

It may take a while for your mind to catch up with your body. You may find yourself trying on much larger sizes than you can actually fit in to. You have a hard time registering when people who haven't seen you in a while look surprised and tell you how great you look. You see the numbers on the scale and look in the mirror and still see the obese you. This is very common and very normal for people to have a delayed reaction in mentally accepting their new bodies. Self-talk really helps during this time, as well as looking at old pictures. You need to say, "I really am ____ pounds. I have lost _____ pounds. I'm thinner and healthier." Always end self-talk with the phrase, "I Love Me." You have probably spent years beating yourself up and undervaluing yourself. You should not allow your weight to define you any more as it has in the past. You are so much more than your outer shell. As you transition in this process, you need to focus on loving yourself as a whole. This means accepting all of you. It's fine to feel accepted by others, but the goal is to accept yourself. As you go through this process, you need to find a balance in being disciplined but being gentle with yourself. You need to become comfortable with giving yourself praise and self-respect. The love and admiration you develop for yourself will produce those long-lasting results because you will be less likely to self-sabotage. Many have difficulty with this as they have focused on caring for others as opposed to themselves for most of their lives. Now suddenly, it seems selfish to focus on yourself first. Let me let you in on a little secret. This is not being selfish; it's called self-preservation. It is imperative to focus on your health in order to be able to care for others' needs. How many times have you told other people to take care of themselves? Why is it so difficult to follow your own advice? Most of the time it's because you hold the role of caregiver. People are used to you taking care of or "fixing things." Now it's time to take care of you first. In doing this, others may say you're acting "different" or "full of yourself." Honestly, all you're doing is finally putting yourself first. Positive affirmations are crucial. To assist with this, making a positive affirmation such as, "I value my ability to make good choices" are important to say each day. To make these affirmations stick, you need to not only say it, but you also need to write it. Particularly if you are a visual learner, you need to see the words. Get in the habit of saying one positive affirmation to yourself each day. Write it on a post-it note. Post it where you will see it—on the mirror, closet door, the refrigerator, or anywhere where you will see it often. After you come to believe one affirmation, move on to another. As simple as it sounds, again it means adopting a routine. This will work if you use it daily. Speak Itit, write it, see it, *be it*!

In this process as you develop life-long positive habits, some other habits may want to creep up as negative coping skills. Be aware that some people have an addiction to food and/or an addictive personality. Be aware of your family history of addiction or developing an addiction to add another outlet that becomes a coping skill. However it comes out, if you are an addict or have a family history, you need to be aware and careful not to substitute food for alcohol, substances, shopping, or gambling. It will always be a struggle to overcome if you have a past history. The more confidence you have in yourself to make better choices, the better chance you have of finding balance post-surgery. Addiction is a pattern of behavior. Just because you may not physically be able to eat, your mind may tell you to continue to eat, making you physically ill, causing dumping syndrome, and ultimately stretching your stomach pouch. Hence feeling sick, increase in vomiting or diarrhea, and the cycle begins again. For many people, although becoming physically ill is a deterrent to food, they find alcohol, shopping, or gambling easy substitutes. Recognize food is everywhere and you need food to survive. Often once the urge to overeat is overcome, those others addictions take over. A very common substitute post-surgery is excess exercise, believe it or not. Although exercise is a very important part of maintaining healthy weight, anything in excess is not healthy physically or mentally. For many people who have lost a significant amount of weight, exercise feels good for the first time. To use all these parts of your body and to feel strong feels great. When those endorphins really kick in, it's very easy to want to maintain that feeling. Not in a rational sense of wanting that energy boost, but the uncontrollable *need* to feel that boost. This is when you need to keep all things in moderation. Ultimately you will set yourself up to fail if you think you can spend three to four hours a day at the gym. This is unrealistic and takes away from other pleasures in your life, like friends and family. You need balance, and spending this much time every day on exercise will present wear and tear on your body over time, as well as your relationships. Forty-five minutes to an hour four to five times per week is plenty to help you reach realistic goals. For maintenance, three to four times a week is sufficient. The point is, there is a difference in using exercise as a diversion to a trigger or to use it to decompress in healthy manner, or to constantly worrying if you can get to the gym equipment for three to four hours at a time. When it becomes obsessive or you become emotional when you miss a workout, examine your motives. If you are giving up time with family and friends every day, it's time to get back to balance. Yes, focus on you first, but balance means having equal parts of physical, social, and emotional well being.

Keep in mind, anything is excess can lead to addiction. I cannot stress this enough. It will do you no good to be thinner only to be addicted to drugs, alcohol, or swimming in debt. I know many people overlook shopping as an addiction, but it can be very easy to get a little too excited to buy a new wardrobe and shop in regular size stores. It's exciting and fun; just don't break the bank in the process. I will be the first one to admit, I think you should get that one pair of jeans you always wanted but could never wear, if you can afford it and stick to one pair. It's when one pair becomes ten and expensive labels outgrow your budget that this becomes an addiction. You may need to enlist the help of others in the process, but you ultimately need to regain control. Control can be had with support and love for yourself. I believe no one wants to harm him or herself, but compulsions and obsessions are powerful monsters. Proper planning is the key. Continue to self evaluate. If you develop an addiction, this is no time for pride. There are support groups for pretty much every addiction. You do need to arm yourself with knowledge and always be prepared for the "what ifs." If you find groups or names of a therapist to assist you if needed ahead of time, you will be ahead of the game. Use your resources. Think about how much courage it took to decide to let someone rearrange your insides. Use that courage to take control in other areas of your life. Every time the urge to go overboard comes, use that positive self-talk, use your faith if you are spiritual, and use your supports. Remember, you are your best friend, no longer your worst enemy. Treat yourself as you would your most cherished loved one. You would never harm him or her, so don't harm yourself by self sabotage. You decided to take charge and live life. Take it for all it is worth.

After reading this, I hope you have a better understanding of all the areas of your life that can be affected post-surgery. I think it's important to at least have an idea of how you can be affected psychologically. You now have the tools you need to combat those uneducated people who say this surgery is a "quick fix." For those who have not done the research or those who have not been through this experience, it appears the weight falls off with little effort. Of course, this is completely untrue. This process takes continual self-evaluation, commitment, and resolve. This process can be life changing in the best of ways and can allow you to experience life with a whole new outlook. If life was good before, it can be great afterward. It can be a lasting solution to better health and add years to your life. Like so many others, I can honestly say this is the best thing I have ever done for myself. It has led me to feel better physically, has increased my energy, and has boosted my self-confidence to a new level. I wish you the best of luck in your journey and remember ... you come first, you deserve to feel good, and above all, changes come from the love you give yourself.

The Journeys

What follows are some true stories of the struggles and success of some of my patients' journeys. I have had the unique opportunity and am so humbled that my patients have chosen to share the details of their journeys with me. These stories are told with each person's permission, with the names and some details changed to protect those who have the courage to share part of their life story with me. These patients recognize that their stories may help to inspire others, acknowledge some issues that are to be addressed, and give others some added insight into their post-surgical experiences.

Take the story of a patient we will refer to as Paige. Paige came to me shortly after her surgery, as she recognized her previous relationship with food was unhealthy and acknowledged her history of emotional eating could be a struggle in the future. Paige had written about her connection with food pre-surgery and said good-bye to her old dear friend. She vowed to change her outlook regarding her relationship with food, her body, and her overall life. Paige was determined, insightful, and willing to do the work to feel whole in mind, body, and spirit. This work also involved Paige changing her relationship with her closest friends and family, including the very co-dependent relationship she had with her mother.

So the happy outcome is Paige followed all the doctors' instructions, lost a ton of weight, and developed a healthy relationship with her mom, right? Actually, these things did happen, but not without a lot of tears (of joy and pain), a lot of both positive and negative feedback, and working out all those old "fat girl" feelings and mentality along the way. Paige would come to session at times tearful because she could see the graze eating patterns of eating resurfacing. She would process her feelings and would recognize her need for immediate gratification and would self sabotage and then beat herself up for entering the cycle. The difference for Paige came when she was able to be more patient with her weight loss and be kinder to herself. She was letting go of the all or none mentality of dieting. She faced many stressors, which affected how she was eating. She struggled to consistently set boundaries with her mother. She began to forgive her father. Paige began the task of dating, and realized she did not have to settle for being second best. She did see the positive qualities she wanted in a relationship, but came to see she needed more, and expressed it. Imagine having the courage to tell your significant other, this is what I need, and if you can't give it to me, I need to move on.

Paige also learned to develop her own sense of style. For the first time, she bought clothes that actually showed off her curves, rather than hiding under clothes that merely helped her to "blend in." Paige learned persistence and patience in many areas of her life, being more gentle and forgiving of herself as time went on. She eliminated those "friends" that hindered her emotionally and began to seek positive people in her life. She learned that only people who could give as well as take belonged in her life. Paige made some career changes, knowing her current job was just not satisfying and willing to take some risk to explore different options. Paige began to really appreciate her body through exercise for the first time and could jog, hop, skip, and run just because it felt good. Paige came to believe in herself. She began to heal physically, emotionally, and spiritually.

Does she still struggle at times? Of course. Paige continues to work on accepting that perfection is not attainable, that only trying her best is good enough each day. Paige is able to waver, as we all do at times, and move forward. She did not do it alone and did not achieve results without feeling drained at times. Life happened and she was able to move through it with a sense of purpose, even in the face of adversity. She became "unstuck." Paige represents all those patients who are fearful of developing a sense of self. She represents the hope that once those fears are met head on, they diminish, and a new, focused, positive person emerges.

Paige was a younger patient, one who had the whole world to explore after twenty-eight years of being trapped in herself. Our next patient's journey happened later in life. We'll call this patient Nina. When Nina came to me for a pre-surgery psychosocial assessment, she could barely walk. She was receiving disability due to severe physical ailments. Nina admitted she was depressed, in a constrictive, controlling marriage of more than thirty years, was unable to be mobile, and truly recognized that bariatric surgery may have been the last chance for obtaining a better quality of life to any degree. Nina was desperate to regain her life. Despite the barriers, she had a wide grin and her openness to follow the protocol and make changes was evident.

Fast forward to Nina fourteen months later. Nina came into the office with that wide smile, had lost more than 130 pounds, and had made all sorts of positive changes in her life. She had left her husband, was working two part-time jobs, applied for first-time home ownership, and attended the gym regularly to sustain her newfound energy. Although Nina used her strong support systems, she was truly on her own for the first time. Nina acknowledged her fears, but used those fears to motivate her to take full advantage of her ability to become active and healthy. Just knowing she took proper steps to become independent also encouraged her to enroll in school part-time in addition to all her other accomplishments. Nina had the support of people who encouraged her and did not make her feel guilty for focusing on herself. Although she at times worried about long-term success, she also knew from her past that as long as she maintains her focus, she can continue to build her life to the fullest.

I would like you to meet Dan. A few years ago Dan was one of a few men that I had worked with who chose to pursue gastric bypass surgery. Now it appears men are much more open to this form of weight loss, and I see nearly as many men as I do women for pre-surgical assessments. I will say it seems men do not follow up on the psychological aspects post-surgery as readily as women, but hopefully that trend will also change with time. Dan came back after losing his weight fairly quickly and began having difficulty in his marriage. Dan also came to recognize he was having difficulty in embracing his new healthy lifestyle, as his wife was unsupportive of his weight loss, which caused mixed emotions for Dan throughout the process. Dan spent quite some time examining his relationship and over time came to realize not only was his wife sabotaging his best efforts, but that her own mental health issues also needed to be addressed. Luckily Dan had other positive support systems in his life and a wonderful relationship with his son to consider. Dan eventually was able to release himself from a destructive relationship with his wife and was able to begin to enjoy all the exciting experiences of becoming healthy and enjoying experiences without the excess weight to hold him back. It took a tremendous amount of courage and insight for Dan to admit that he had not caused his relationship to dissolve. He was able to admit the relationship initially stemmed from Dan receiving attention, even if the attention was negative. Over time Dan began to develop the self-confidence to allow himself to desire a more positive relationship and let go of the fear of being alone and did not settle for negative attention being acceptable. Once again, fear can be a powerful motivator to stay in a destructive relationship or a motivator to make some difficult changes. Through self-analysis, Dan was able to focus on his positive qualities and embrace those small but exciting changes, like having more energy to be more active, without feeling guilty for taking care of himself first before caring for others' needs. This caretaker mentality can sabotage the best of intentions if you do not learn to change your thinking for self-preservation as opposed to being self-involved. It really is okay to look out for your needs first in any relationship, as long as the give and take is fairly equitable.

I would like to introduce you to Tia. Tia is witty, attractive, and has a great sense of humor. Outwardly, Tia appears to be pretty self-confident. In reality, Tia has a bad habit of not feeling "good enough" and has some unresolved issues with her "fat girl" mentality, which has made for a difficult road for Tia to truly appreciate her new self. Although Tia lost over one hundred pounds, medical issues keep her from attaining her goal weight and added to her feeling frustrated with accepting what she had accomplished, as opposed to obsessing on what was yet to come. In addition, issues of dating for the first time in several years, becoming comfortable with her sexuality, avoiding sabotaging relationships, finding satisfying career goals, and overall not feeling satisfied with herself were issues Tia struggled with in our time together. At times, Tia was so discouraged that depression took over and she could really not see all she had achieved. Tia did take advantage of her resources, used all her wonderful supports, and eventually began to make some changes. Despite her fear of rejection, Tia had the courage to begin to date again, started to reconnect with her sexuality, allowed herself to become more emotionally connected to others, chose to return to school to jumpstart her career, and began to put her medical issues in perspective. Did I say Tia is what we call a "Type A" personality? She is very much a perfectionist and gets stuck in all good or all bad thinking. Her struggle was more difficult, as she needed to allow herself some room and some patience in accepting the reality of her situation. There is no perfect way to behave each day. She still struggles with issues of self-esteem (really, who does not), but has allowed herself to be open to some experiences that have allowed her to feel on a deeper level. Scary but necessary. This is all to say that issues may never disappear, but they can be put into perspective and worked on as you work on becoming happy and healthy.

Then there was Shashi. Shashi had a magnetic personality and a wonderful compassion for others. Unfortunately, as Shashi has suffered some severe trauma in her life and continued to struggle with an eating disorder, she had difficulty having compassion for herself. Shashi could not see the seventy-pound weight loss she had achieved and had great difficultly disconnecting emotionally from food. She was wise enough to seek professional help in many areas to assist her in her journey. Shashi did use her bariatric supports, as well as the support of her family and friends. At times, Shashi needed to disengage herself from toxic people in her life, always having a difficult time breaking ties. Shashi does a great job with keeping up with exercise, and even can give herself credit in this area at times. Shashi's biggest obstacle is her lack of self-worth, and her tendency to compare herself with others, always selling herself short. Today, Shashi continues to evolve in the process, often using her resources and riding a positive wave, other times self-sabotaging her best efforts. The roller coaster ride continues, but if Shashi continues to work on issues of self-esteem and resolving some deeper past issues, she will continue to become an overall healthier person. I feel it's important to share Shashi's journey to point out the successes along with the struggles. It is so easy to beat ourselves down, and so much harder to build ourselves up. While it would be wonderful to say all stories after gastric bypass end in success without struggle, this would be unfair and misleading. Shashi's story reminds us that we will always have life issues to deal with, and food can be a detrimental coping skill. This needs to be acknowledged in order to replace it with other coping mechanisms that are positive and add to a better quality of life.

I could go on for endless pages reveling in the various journeys I have had the privilege of witnessing over the past few years. Hopefully through this book you have found different aspects that you can identify with, and others that have sparked your consideration in your journey. It is my hope these words will serve as an additional tool that you can come back to periodically should you face the psychological aspects of your journey, and hopefully inspire you to explore your world in new and exciting ways. Above all, be kind to yourself, take advantage of all the new and wonderful experiences you may face, and sit back and contemplate your own journey. Allow your world to expand to include positive supports, and remember you are not alone in this journey to become healthy and whole.